NOURISHING YOUR PREGNANCY DIET COOKBOOK

A Comprehensive Guide to Healthy Eating for Expecting Moms

Adam C.

ISBN: 9798864523766

DEDICATION

This book is dedicated to all my Readers

CONTENTS

Introduction

Welcome to the "Nourishing Your Pregnancy Diet Cookbook: A Comprehensive Guide to Healthy Eating for Expecting Moms."

Concerning This Cookbook

The journey of pregnancy is amazing, full of transformation, joy, and anticipation. The body goes through amazing changes during this time in order to nurture and promote the development of a new life. During this time, nutrition is crucial to the health and wellbeing of both mother and child. This cookbook is intended to be your dependable travel partner on this meaningful journey. It provides a multitude of meal planning, recipes, and advice to support you in making wholesome decisions during your pregnancy.

The Value of Nutrition throughout Pregnancy

It's important to eat healthily for two during pregnancy rather than just eating for two. During pregnancy, your body need more nutrients, and the appropriate meals can help your unborn child's key organs, brain, and general health develop. Additionally, a well-balanced diet can improve your mood, ease typical pregnant discomforts, and get your body ready for labor and postpartum recovery.

The future health and wellbeing of your unborn kid is significantly impacted by what you consume while pregnant. That's why we wrote this cookbook: to arm you with information, entice you with scrumptious dishes, and provide you the means to choose what's best for you and your unborn child.

Uses for This Book

For the best use of "Nourishing Your Pregnancy Diet Cookbook," we advise beginning with a careful reading of the chapter's introduction to pregnancy nutrition. This will give you a clear idea of the vital nutrients your body requires and how important they are to the growth of your child.

Examine the meal-planning examples in Chapter 2, which are specific to each trimester. You can use these as a starting point for your own meal planning to make sure you get the right nutrients at the right times during your pregnancy.

Then, go through the book's chapters, each of which is brimming with delectable, nutrient-dense dishes created especially for expectant mothers. You can quickly find options for breakfast, lunch, supper, snacks, and even postpartum meals thanks to the organization of the recipes by meal type.

Additionally, Chapter 8 contains a section on special dietary considerations that covers a variety of dietary preferences and limits. You'll find advice and recipes that are tailored to your particular requirements, whether you're a vegetarian, vegan, or need gluten-free options.

You can find more informational sources, meal planning templates, and useful reading materials to further your understanding of pregnancy nutrition in the appendix.

Our aim is to make your pregnancy experience little simpler, much healthier, and thoroughly pleasant. You'll be better able to enjoy the magic of pregnancy and secure a healthy start for your expanding family if you nourish your body with the appropriate foods. We hope that this cookbook proves to be a priceless ally in your journey to a healthy and happy pregnancy.

Chapter 1: Understanding Pregnancy Nutrition

A time of great change and transition is pregnancy. Your body is producing the ideal conditions for a new life to thrive and flourish in addition to sustaining itself. Understanding the pillars of pregnancy nutrition is essential before beginning this amazing adventure.

1.1 Requirements for Nutrition during Pregnancy

Your nutritional requirements rise throughout pregnancy to support both your health and the development of your unborn child. Consuming a diet that is well-balanced and rich in a range of nutrients is crucial to meeting these objectives. The essential nutrients you'll require are summarized here:

- **Folic acid:** is a B-vitamin that is crucial for embryonic development in the early stages and can guard against neural tube abnormalities. Citrus fruits, leafy greens, and fortified cereals all contain it.

- **Iron:** Iron is essential for both avoiding anemia and delivering oxygen to your unborn child. Lean meats, legumes, and fortified cereals are excellent sources.

- **Calcium:** Your infant needs calcium to have strong bones and teeth. Leafy greens, fortified plant-based milk, and dairy products are all great sources of calcium.

- **Protein:** The development of your baby's organs and tissues depends on protein. Include lean meats, poultry, fish, eggs, and supplies from plants, such as beans and tofu.

- **Fiber:** Fiber improves digestion and relieves common pregnant aches and pains including constipation. Fiber is abundant in whole grains, fruits, and vegetables.

- **Omega-3 Fatty Acids:** These good fats aid in the growth of your child's brain and eyes. Walnuts, flaxseeds, and fatty fish are excellent sources.

- **Vitamin D:** Vitamin D is necessary for bone health and calcium absorption. This vitamin can be obtained from fortified meals and sun exposure.

- **Vitamin C:** It boosts your immune system and helps the body absorb iron. Vitamin C is abundant in bell peppers, strawberries, and citrus fruits.

- **Vitamin A:** During the early stages of development, this vitamin is essential for your baby's growth. Vitamin A is found in spinach, carrots, and sweet potatoes.

- **Vitamin B12:** Red blood cell formation and neuronal function both benefit from vitamin B12. Since it is mostly present in animal products, vegans should think about taking supplements.

1.2 The Foundation of a Healthful Diet

A balanced pregnancy diet should include a range of foods, each of which has a specialized function. Here are the components of a wholesome diet for expectant mothers:

- Proteins: Proteins are necessary for the growth and development of your infant. Include lean sources of protein in your meals, such as beans, tofu, and lean meats, chicken, fish, and eggs.

- Fruits and vegetables: These are excellent sources of fiber, vitamins, and minerals. A wide range of nutrients are ensured by a vivid diversity.

- Complex carbs, fiber, and vital nutrients are found in whole grains including brown rice, quinoa, and whole-grain bread.

- Dairy and dairy substitutes are good sources of calcium and vitamin D for healthy bones and teeth. When possible, use low-fat or plant-based solutions.

- Omega-3 fatty acids, which are present in foods like fatty fish, flaxseed, and walnuts, enhance your baby's brain development.

- Staying properly hydrated is essential because dehydration can cause problems. The best options are water, herbal teas, and diluted fruit juices.

1.3 Essential Vitamins and Minerals for Pregnant Women

To preserve the health of both themselves and their unborn children, pregnant women need to consume more of some vitamins and minerals. Let's examine some of the major actors in more detail:

- Folic acid, often known as folate, is crucial during the first trimester of pregnancy. It promotes the growth of the baby's nervous system and aids in the prevention of neural tube abnormalities.

- Iron: Iron is essential for your blood to carry oxygen to your unborn child. Additionally, it helps your body's increased blood volume while you're pregnant.

- Calcium: Calcium is essential for the growth of your baby's bones and teeth as well as for maintaining the health of your own bones.

- Vitamin D: Vitamin D is necessary for the growth of your baby's bones and aids in the body's absorption of calcium.

- Vitamin C: Vitamin C boosts your immune system at this crucial period and helps the body absorb iron.

- Vitamin A: Vitamin A is crucial for the growth and maturation of your baby's immune system.

- Vitamin B12: Vitamin B12 is essential for the development of red blood cells and neurological function.

- Omega-3 Fatty Acids: Your baby's brain and eyes develop significantly in response to these good fats.

1.4 Dietary Special Considerations

Every pregnancy is different, and every person's nutritional requirements may be different. There may be specific dietary needs for some women, such as:

- Diets that are vegetarian or vegan require special attention to supplies of iron, vitamin B12, and protein that come from plant-based meals and supplements.

- Gluten-free diets: If you have celiac disease or gluten intolerance, choosing gluten-free grains like rice, quinoa, and corn will help you have a safe pregnancy.

- Women who have gestational diabetes must carefully control their carbohydrate intake and blood sugar levels. Making an appropriate food plan can be assisted by a nutritionist.

- Food Allergies: If you have a food allergy, make sure your pregnancy diet is allergen-free and has suitable replacements.

Your road to comprehending and handling pregnancy nutrition doesn't end with this chapter. We'll go into detail about meal planning, recipes, and other factors in the chapters that follow to help you efficiently eat for both your body and your developing baby. Remember that every pregnancy is different, so it's always a good idea to seek professional advice from a certified dietitian or healthcare professional.

Chapter 2: Planning Your Meals for a Healthy Pregnancy

One of the most crucial things you can do to make sure you and your unborn child receive the vital nutrients required for a healthy and happy pregnancy is to create a well-balanced pregnancy food plan. We'll delve into the art of meal planning in this chapter and look at how to respond to the special opportunities and challenges that each trimester offers.

2.1 Making a Balanced Meal Plan for Pregnancy

When planning your meals during pregnancy, make sure to choose a variety of foods that offer the proper amounts of the essential nutrients. Here are some important guidelines to bear in mind:

- Incorporate a variety of food groups into your diet, such as fruits, vegetables, whole grains, lean proteins, and dairy or dairy substitutes. This variety will make it easier for you to consume all of the necessary nutrients.

- Portion Control: Although you require more calories during pregnant, it's crucial to keep your intake in check. Make every food count during pregnancy rather than indulging excessively.

- Eating regular meals and snacks can help control blood sugar levels and ease common pregnant discomforts like nausea and heartburn.

- Hydration: It's important to maintain proper hydration. At least 8 to 10 cups of water should be consumed every day. You can also want to add herbal teas and diluted fruit juices.

- Supplements: Talk to your doctor to see whether you need to take any special supplements, including prenatal vitamins, to make up for any nutritional shortfalls.

2.2 Sample Menus for Every Trimester

Your nutrient needs will fluctuate as the pregnancy goes on. Here are some examples of meal plans for each stage of pregnancy to help you understand how to modify your diet.

Weeks 1–12 of the first trimester

You can feel drained and morning ill throughout the first trimester. Focusing on bland, simple-to-digest foods are essential. A first trimester meal plan example is shown below:

Breakfast:

- Few berries, honey, and plain Greek yogurt

- Toast made of whole grains and almond butter

Lunch:

- Grilled chicken or a plant-based protein in a mixed green salad

- Whole-grain crackers as a side dish

Dinner:

- A tofu stir-fry with lots of vegetables or baked salmon

- Brown rice or quinoa as a side dish

Snacks:

- Banana or apple slices with almond or peanut butter

- Several nuts for an increase in protein

Weeks 13–27 of the second trimester

The nausea frequently goes away and your energy levels rise during the second trimester. It's a great idea to add more ethnic foods now:

Breakfast:

- Breakfast of scrambled eggs, whole-grain bread, and spinach
- Freshly squeezed orange juice in a glass

Lunch:

- Avocado and lime vinaigrette on top of a quinoa and black bean salad
- Whole-grain crackers as a side dish

Dinner:

- A lentil stew with a variety of veggies or grilled shrimp
- Sweet potatoes or wild rice mashed

Snacks:

- Greek yogurt accompanied by oats and fruit.

- Hummus and carrot and cucumber sticks

Weeks 28–40 of the third trimester

You can have heartburn and a bigger appetite as the third trimester approaches. It's critical to control portion sizes and select foods that are easy on the stomach:

Breakfast:

- Oatmeal with banana slices and honey drizzle
- A cup of milk or plant-based milk with added nutrients

Lunch:

- A wrap made of turkey or tempeh and loaded with vegetables
- An appetizer salad

Dinner:

- Steamed broccoli with baked chicken or a chickpea curry as a side dish

- Whole-grain pasta or quinoa

Snacks:

- Cottage cheese and pineapple, fresh

2.3 A few almonds to boost your energy adapting to Pregnancy Symptoms

It's critical to understand that no two pregnancies are the same. Common symptoms that may have an impact on your eating patterns include morning sickness, food aversions, and cravings. Here are some suggestions for handling these signs:

- Try eating small, frequent meals and concentrating on bland, easily digestible foods like crackers, bread, and clear broths if morning sickness is a problem.

- Food aversions: Look for alternate sources of the same nutrients if particular foods make you nauseous. Consider fortified plant-based milk if you can't tolerate dairy, for instance, if you need calcium.

- Cravings: You should periodically give into your cravings, but attempt to counteract them with nutrient-dense foods. If you have a sweet tooth, think about fruit or yogurt with honey.

- Avoid consuming heavy meals, especially in the evening, to control heartburn. Choose smaller, more frequent meals, and stay away from hot or acidic foods.

As your pregnancy develops, keep in mind that adaptability is essential. Depending on how you're feeling, you might need to change your food plans. A certified dietician or your healthcare practitioner should always be consulted for tailored guidance and to address any particular dietary problems. Through careful food preparation and flexibility, you can hydrate both your body and your developing baby during this amazing journey.

Chapter 3: Breakfast treats

Breakfast is frequently regarded as the most significant meal of the day, and during pregnancy, this is especially true. It jump-starts your metabolism, gives you energy for the day, and aids with blood sugar stabilization. To make sure you start your day off right, we'll look at a variety of nutrient-dense morning meals in this chapter, from invigorating smoothies and shakes to filling breakfast bowls and on-the-go options.

3.1 Nutrient-dense breakfasts

A healthy meal is a fantastic chance to provide your body and developing baby the nutrients it needs. When making your breakfast, bear in mind the following important nutrients:

1. Protein: Protein supports the growth of the organs and tissues in your unborn child. Lean meats, dairy products, eggs, lentils, and plant-based protein sources like tofu should all be included in your breakfast.

2. Constipation and other common pregnant discomforts can be eased with fiber, which also helps with digestion. Excellent

sources include fruits, whole grains, and veggies.

3. Calcium: Calcium is crucial for both the growth of your baby's bones and the preservation of your own bone health. Include dairy or dairy substitutes with added vitamins in your morning meal.

4. During the first trimester of pregnancy, folate is essential for preventing neural tube abnormalities. Leafy greens, citrus fruits, and fortified cereals all contain folate.

5. Omega-3 Fatty Acids: These good fats aid in the growth of your child's brain and eyes. Think about including fatty salmon, chia seeds, or flaxseeds in your breakfast.

3.2 Energizing Shakes and smoothies

Smoothies and shakes are a tasty and practical way to include a variety of nutrients in one meal. Following are a few suggestions for revitalizing morning blends:

1. *Berry Blast Smoothie*

Greek yogurt, assorted berries, a banana, and some honey are all combined in a blender. Protein, antioxidants, and a touch of sweetness come naturally in this smoothie.

2. Green Goddess Shake

Combine banana, Greek yogurt, kale, spinach, and a few almonds. This protein-, vitamin-, and mineral-rich green smoothie

3. Protein shake with chocolate and peanut butter

For a filling and invigorating shake, mix unsweetened cocoa powder, peanut butter, protein powder, and banana with milk or a dairy substitute.

4. Smoothie with Tropical Delight

Combine coconut milk, mango, pineapple, and a hint of vanilla. This smoothie provides important vitamins as well as a flavor of the tropics.

3.3 Full-bodied breakfast bowls

Breakfast bowls let you blend a variety of nutrient-dense ingredients while also being aesthetically pleasing. Following are some recipes for filling breakfast bowls:

1. *Oats with Berries Overnight*

The night before, make oats with almond milk and chia seeds. Fresh berries, honey, and a garnish of chopped almonds should be added on top.

2. *A bowl of breakfast quinoa*

Sliced bananas, chopped almonds, and a dollop of Greek yogurt are added to cooked quinoa. Add honey for additional sweetness.

3. *Pudding made with chia seeds*

Chia seeds should be combined with milk and refrigerated overnight. Add granola, cut fruit, and a sprinkle of cinnamon on top in the morning.

4. *A Greek yogurt parfait*

Strawberries cut into slices, granola, and maple syrup are all layered on top of Greek yogurt. This bowl is calcium and protein-rich.

3.4 Mobile Options

The following are some wholesome on-the-go breakfast options for those hectic mornings when you need something quick and portable:

1. *Burrito for breakfast*

Wrap a whole-grain tortilla around scrambled eggs, black beans, and salsa. It is a portable choice that is high in protein.

2. *Banana and Nut Butter Sandwich*

Sliced banana and almond or peanut butter on whole-grain toast make a filling and portable breakfast

3. *Energy Snacks*

Prepare oat, honey, nut, and dried fruit energy bites. They are ideal for munching on while traveling.

4. *Muffins with high fiber*

Make a batch of fruit-, whole-grain-, and bran-filled muffins. These can be prepared in advance and picked up as you leave.

A nutrient-rich breakfast lays the foundation for a healthy day during your pregnancy. Whether you have time for a leisurely morning meal or need something quick and portable, there are lots of alternatives to help you jumpstart your day with the nourishment both you and your baby need.

Chapter 4: Filling Lunches

During pregnancy, lunch provides a chance to refresh your body with necessary nutrients. It's important to choose healthful food choices that are also delicious. We'll look at a variety of lunch alternatives in this chapter, including easy and filling salads, flavorful sandwiches and wraps, protein-rich soups and stews, and quick, wholesome meals that can be made in no time.

4.1 Simple Salads That Are Filling

Salads are a great lunchtime option for including a range of veggies, proteins, and healthy fats. Here are some suggestions for quick and filling salads:

1. *Salad of spinach and strawberries*

Sliced strawberries, feta cheese, and a few walnuts should all be added to fresh spinach. Balsamic vinaigrette should be drizzled for a sweet and savory salad.

2. *Greek Salad*

Combine tomatoes, cucumbers, olives, feta cheese, and red onion to make a Greek salad, for more protein, top with grilled chicken or chickpeas.

3. *Caprese salad*

Slices of fresh mozzarella, basil leaves, and tomato are layered. For a delicious salad with an Italian flair, drizzle with balsamic glaze and extra virgin olive oil.

4. *Salad with roasted vegetables and quinoa*

Combine cooked quinoa with your preferred vegetables once they have been roasted. For a tasty and healthy dinner, add some lemon juice and olive oil.

4.2 Savory wraps and Sandwiches

A quick and portable lunch choice is a sandwich or a wrap. For savory fillings, consider the following:

1. Sandwich with turkey and avocado:

For a filling sandwich, spread avocado over whole-grain bread and top with lean turkey, lettuce, and tomato.

2. Wrap with hummus and vegetables:

Spread hummus on a whole grain tortilla, then top with spinach, red pepper strips, and cucumber slices. For a quick and wholesome meal, roll it up.

3. A sandwich with tuna salad:

Combine Greek yogurt or mayonnaise, diced pickles, and a touch of mustard with canned tuna. Spread on whole-wheat bread, and then add lettuce and tomato on top.

4. The Caprese Wrap

A whole-grain tortilla should be used to encase tomato slices, mozzarella, and basil leaves. Roll it up and drizzle it with balsamic glaze for a delectable and healthy meal.

4.3 Rich in Protein Soups and Stews

In addition to being warming, soups and stews are also a fantastic source of protein and vitamins. Here are some possibilities for a filling lunch that are high in protein:

1. lentil soup

Protein and fiber are abundant in lentil soup. For added taste, include veggies and a variety of seasonings.

2. Stew with chicken and vegetables:

Lean chicken, a variety of veggies, and flavorful herbs and spices make a filling stew.

3. Soup with black beans:

Protein-rich black bean soup can be spiced up with chili powder and finished with Greek yogurt for a creamy appearance.

4. Soup with quinoa and vegetables:

To provide more protein, add quinoa to a vegetable soup. To receive the most nutrients, choose a range of colored vegetables.

4.4 Fast and wholesome lunches

Quick and wholesome lunches can save the day when time is of the essence. Here are some suggestions for quick-to-prepare meals:

1. Stir-Fried vegetables:

Tofu, chicken, and a variety of colorful veggies are stir-fried in teriyaki or soy sauce. For a quick, nutrient-rich lunch, serve over brown rice.

2. Egg salad:

Hard-boiled eggs can be combined with Greek yogurt, mustard, and finely sliced green onions to make an easy egg salad. Serve with whole-grain bread or crackers.

3. Toast with avocado:

For a quick and wholesome meal, spread avocado over whole-wheat toast and top with salt, red pepper flakes, and olive oil.

4. Remainings:

Don't forget about dinner from yesterday night. The next day's lunch can frequently be made with excellent, time-saving, and fulfilling leftovers.

Lunches should be enjoyable and nourishing when you're pregnant. There are numerous ways to make certain that you and your developing baby are receiving the crucial nutrients needed for a healthy and bright pregnancy, whether you choose salads, sandwiches, soups, or quick and healthy options.

Chapter 5: A Couple's Dinner

Dinner is the ideal chance to have a satisfying and comfortable meal with your developing child as the day comes to an end. In this chapter, we look at a range of supper options made specifically for expectant mothers, such as one-pan wonders for convenience, hearty casseroles and bakes, international cuisines to entice your palate, and vegetarian and vegan meal options for people with specific dietary needs.

5.1 Single-Item Wonders

One-pan meals make it simple to prepare an evening meal that is both wholesome and balanced. Some one-pan wonders are listed below:

1. Salmon on a sheet pan with roasted vegetables

On a sheet pan, arrange a variety of bright veggies around the salmon fillets, drizzle the dish with olive oil and your preferred seasonings.

2. Chicken with lemon and garlic and asparagus

Fresh asparagus and chicken breasts are baked together with a tangy lemon-garlic sauce drizzled over them for flavor.

3. Baked vegetables with sausage:

For a filling and savory dinner, combine sausage, bell peppers, onions, and zucchini on a sheet pan.

4. Stir-Fry with Quinoa and Vegetables:

To prepare quinoa stir-fry, combine quinoa with a variety of stir-fried vegetables, tofu, and a flavorful sauce in a big skillet.

5.2 Comforting Bakes & Casseroles

Baked goods and casseroles provide a warm, cozy method to sate your appetite and nourish your body. Here are some soothing suggestions:

1. Chicken pot pie casserole, to start:

Lean chicken, mixed veggies, and a creamy sauce should be combined to make a chicken pot pie filling. A flaky pastry crust should then be placed on top.

2. Enchiladas with sweet potatoes and black beans

Sweet potato and black bean enchiladas with a spicy sauce and cheese make a tasty and wholesome meal.

3. Ziti Baked:

Use whole-grain pasta, lean ground beef or turkey, lots of vegetables, and a rich tomato sauce to make baked ziti.

4. Eggplant Parmigiana:

Layers of breaded and baked eggplant pieces, marinara sauce, and mozzarella cheese provide a hearty, meatless choice.

5.3 International Cuisine for Moms-to-Be

Your food during pregnancy might be excitingly flavored by experimenting with different cuisines. Here are some meal ideas with an international flair:

1. Tofu and Thai Red Curry

Tofu, veggies, and fragrant herbs combine to create a Thai red curry dish that is robust and spicy.

2. Tagine of Moroccan chickpeas:

Try a flavorful chickpea tagine made with spices, apricots, and soft veggies to experience North African cuisine.

3. Greek Pepper Stuffed:

Fill bell peppers with a mixture of ground lamb or beef, rice, tomatoes, and flavorful herbs to experience Greek flavors.

4. Salmon Teriyaki in Japan:

Steamed jasmine rice, sautéed bok choy, and teriyaki fish in the style of Japanese cuisine will satisfy your cravings.

5.4 Dinner options for vegetarians and vegans

Here are some wholesome and delectable meal suggestions for individuals who follow a vegetarian or vegan diet:

1. Lasagna with butternut squash and spinach

Layer roasted butternut squash, sautéed spinach, and a rich béchamel sauce to make vegetarian lasagna.

2. Curry with Lentils and Vegetables:

With lentils, a variety of veggies, and a variety of fragrant spices, you can make a delicious vegan curry.

3. Steaks with portobello mushrooms:

For a filling vegan supper, grill or roast portobello mushrooms with a flavorful marinade.

4. Shawarma with cauliflower and chickpeas:

Enjoy a shawarma of cauliflower and chickpeas with tahini sauce and warm pita bread to experience the tastes of the Middle East.

While enjoying a range of delicious and healthy dishes, dinnertime during pregnancy can be an opportunity to strengthen your relationship with your developing child. Whether you choose one-pan meals, hearty casseroles, exotic cuisines, or vegetarian and vegan options, the important thing is to eat meals that nourish your body and sate your cravings.

Chapter 6: Snacks and Sides

In your pregnancy diet, snacks and side dishes can be crucial since they provide you the chance to give your body the nutrition it needs, fulfill cravings, and keep your energy levels stable. We'll look at a range of options in this chapter, including nutrient-dense snacks, delectable dips and spreads, filling side dishes, and even healthful sweet treats to indulge in.

6.1 Veggie-Rich Snacking

Snacking throughout pregnancy helps you fill the time between meals, keeping you energized and preventing hunger. Choose nutrient-dense snacks to make sure you and your child get the vitamins and minerals you need. Here are a few concepts:

1. Berries with Greek yogurt:

Greek yogurt is a good source of calcium and protein. Fresh berries on top will add fiber and antioxidants to the dish.

2. Banana and nut butter:

Banana slices should be covered in almond or peanut butter. This snack contains potassium, good fats, and protein.

3. Pineapple with Cottage Cheese:

A powerhouse of protein is cottage cheese. Make a pleasant and calcium-rich snack out of it by serving it with fresh pineapple.

4. Baby carrots and hummus

A fantastic source of plant-based protein is hummus. Baby carrots dipped make a crisp, wholesome snack.

6.2 Scrumptious Spreads and Dips

Your snacks and side dishes might taste better when you use dips and spreads. Here are some suggestions for delectable spreads and dips:

1. Avocado:

Blend tomatoes, onions, cilantro, lime juice, and a little salt with ripe avocados. Serve with sliced vegetables or whole-grain chips.

2. Tzatziki

Combine Greek yogurt, cucumber, garlic, and dill to make

tzatziki. It makes a cool dip for pita bread or sliced cucumbers.

3. Salsa:

With tomatoes, onions, jalapenos, and cilantro, make a fresh salsa. It makes a tangy topping for grilled chicken or fish as well as a zesty addition to tortilla chips.

4. Baba Ghanoush

For a dip with a Mediterranean flavor, roast eggplant, peel it, and then combine it with tahini, garlic, lemon juice, and olive oil.

6.3 Delicious Side Dishes

A simple dinner can become a more satisfying and substantial one with the addition of sides. Here are some suggestions for filling sides:

1. Roasted sweet potatoes:

With a sprinkle of olive oil, salt, and your preferred seasonings, roast sweet potato wedges. These are vitamin and fiber-rich.

2. Quinoa Salad:

Make a beautiful quinoa salad with cucumbers, cherry tomatoes, bell peppers, and zingy vinaigrette.

3. Steaming broccoli with butter and garlic:

For a quick and wholesome side dish, steam broccoli until it is soft and then combines with a garlic butter sauce.

4. Corn on the Cob Grilled:

For a delicious side, grill corn on the cob with a dash of chili powder and a squeeze of lime.

6.4 Wholesome sweet treats

It might be a lovely method to satiate pregnant desires to indulge in a sweet treat. Here are some possibilities for more nutritious sweets:

1. Salad of fruit:

Make a fruit salad by combining a range of vibrant and fresh fruits. For more sweetness, drizzle with honey or sprinkle with cinnamon.

2. Berries with Dark Chocolate Coating:

Dark chocolate can be used to coat strawberries, blueberries, or raspberries for a sweet and anti-oxidant-rich treat.

3. Bark made of frozen yogurt

Greek yogurt should be spread out on a baking sheet. Fruits and honey should be added before freezing. Cut into pieces for a refreshing and filling snack.

4. Baked Apples:

Apples should be cored, filled with a combination of oats, cinnamon, and a little honey, and baked until soft.

You can fuel your body, sate cravings, and keep your energy levels up throughout the day by eating snacks and sides. Whether you choose nutrient-dense snacks, delectable dips and spreads, filling side dishes, or healthier sweet treats, these choices make sure that both you and your unborn child obtain vital nutrients and enjoy the experience of pregnancy.

Chapter 7: Pregnancy and Food Safety

Food safety during pregnancy must be ensured at all costs. Preventing dangerous foodborne infections from harming you and your developing child is a vital part of keeping your pregnancy healthy. This chapter will cover proper food handling and storage techniques, list foods to stay away from while pregnant, and go through how to deal with those inescapable food cravings in a way that puts your health first.

7.1 Managing and Storing Food Safely

A healthy pregnancy requires proper food handling and storage practices. Following are some suggestions:

1. Cleanliness is Important:

Before handling food, wash your hands well, especially if you just handled raw fish, poultry, or meat. To clean kitchen countertops, cutting boards, and cutlery, use hot, soapy water.

2. Keep Cross-Contamination at Bay:

To avoid contamination, keep raw and cooked items apart. For raw meats and veggies, use different chopping boards and utensils.

3. Appropriate Cooling:

Meat, dairy, and leftovers should be kept in the refrigerator at or below 40°F (4°C). Within two hours of preparation, store prepared items in the refrigerator or freezer.

4. Observe the Use-By dates:

To maintain freshness and safety, pay close attention to the use-by dates on food packages and strictly abide by them.

5. Prepare Food Fully:

To get rid of dangerous bacteria, cook meat, poultry, and shellfish to the recommended internal temperatures. To ensure the appropriate temperature, use a food thermometer.

6. Safely Reheat:

To guarantee that all bacteria are eliminated, reheat leftovers to a minimum temperature of 165°F (74°C).

7.2 Foods to Stay away from when Pregnant

While there are many delectable foods to eat while pregnant, it's also important to be aware of foods that should be avoided because of potential dangers. These consist of:

1. Seafood and shellfish that is raw or undercooked:

Because eating raw or undercooked seafood increases your risk of contracting a foodborne disease, it's better to steer clear of sushi, oysters, and other meals of the sort while you're expecting.

2. Dairy products without pasteurization:

Hazardous bacteria can be present in unpasteurized milk, cheese, and other dairy products. Choose pasteurized substitutes to lower the risk.

3. Uncooked or raw eggs:

Salmonella can be present in raw or undercooked eggs, such as those found in homemade Caesar dressing, aioli, or unbaked cookie dough.

4. Preserved Pâté and Deli Meats:

Listeria is a bacterium that can be found in unpasteurized pâté and deli meats, putting both you and your unborn child at danger.

5. Fish High in Mercury:

High mercury levels in some fish, including shark, swordfish, and king mackerel, can be detrimental to embryonic development. Choose low-mercury seafood such as salmon or shrimp.

6. Too much caffeine

Preterm birth and miscarriage risk are both increased by excessive caffeine consumption. You should moderately limit your daily caffeine intake to no more than 200–300 milligrams.

7.3 How to Manage Your Food Cravings

Extreme food cravings are a common side effect of pregnancy. Even if treating yourself once in a while is acceptable, it's crucial to do it in a way that preserves a balanced diet and adheres to safe food standards. Here are some suggestions for controlling your appetite:

1. Use Moderation:

Enjoy your appetites in moderation to prevent them from dominating your diet.

2. Opt for Healthier Substitutions:

Choose some fresh fruit or a little piece of dark chocolate if you're seeking sweets. Pick unsalted nuts or whole-grain crackers to satisfy your desires for salt.

3. Balance with Foods High in Nutrients:

In order to make sure that you are reaching your nutritional needs, satisfy your cravings while balancing them with nutrient-rich foods.

4. Talk to Your Healthcare Professional:

Discuss your cravings with your healthcare practitioner if they are persistent or for un healthful foods, as they may have advice or recommendations regarding nutrition.

You may maintain a healthy diet during your pregnancy by adhering to safe food handling and storage procedures, being aware of items to avoid while pregnant and controlling food cravings in a balanced way. The ultimate objective is to put your health and the welfare of your developing child first.

Chapter 8: Special Dietary Needs

Every woman's experience during pregnancy is different, and her nutritional requirements may change dramatically. In this chapter, we'll discuss special dietary issues that might come up during pregnancy, such as options for those who follow gluten-free or allergen-friendly eating patterns, vegetarian and vegan diets, and gestational diabetes management plans with a diet-specific focus.

8.1 Pregnant Vegetarians and Vegans

It is totally possible to follow a vegetarian or vegan diet while expecting and yet acquire the nutrients you and your baby need. Here are some things to think about:

1. Sources of protein

Dairy, eggs, and plant-based sources of protein including tofu, beans, and nuts are essential for vegetarians. For vegans, fortified foods, plant-based proteins, and maybe B12 and iron supplements are the best options.

2. Calcium Consumption

Calcium can be found in dairy substitutes like tofu, fortified plant-based milk, and leafy greens. Make sure you fulfill your everyday obligations.

3. Foods High in Iron:

Excellent sources of iron include legumes, fortified cereals, and dark leafy greens. Iron absorption is improved when they are combined with foods high in vitamin C.

4. Omega-3 Fatty Acids:

For crucial omega-3 fatty acids, think about plant-based sources like flaxseeds, chia seeds, and walnuts.

5. B12 vitamin:

Vegans should think about taking a B12 supplement because it is mostly found in animal products, although vegetarians can acquire B12 from dairy and eggs.

8.2 Options that are both allergen- and gluten-free

While those with other allergies may take steps to avoid allergens, pregnant people with gluten sensitivities or allergy must maintain a gluten-free diet. Here are some things to think about:

1. Alternatives to Gluten:

Pick grains like quinoa, rice, and oats that are gluten-free. Verify the gluten-free label on packaged items.

2. Alternatives those are Allergen-Friendly:

Look for alternate sources of protein and nutrients if you are allergic to things like nuts or soy.

3. Carefully Read Labels:

Read food labels carefully to spot any potential allergens, and think about buying brands that are allergen-free.

4. Speak with a dietitian or allergist:

Consult a dietician or allergist if you have food sensitivities or allergies to make sure you get the nutrition you need throughout pregnancy.

8.3 Dietary Management of Gestational Diabetes

Dietary decisions are crucial in the management of gestational diabetes, a condition that can arise during pregnancy. The following are some diet tips:

1. Management of Carbohydrates:

To assist in regulating blood sugar levels, place an emphasis on complex carbs, such as whole grains and legumes.

2. Portion Management:

To prevent significant changes in blood sugar, keep an eye on portion sizes. It may be advantageous to consume smaller, more frequent meals.

3. A balanced diet:

Make sure to include lean proteins, healthy fats, and foods high in fiber in your meals to keep they balanced.

4. Observing blood sugar levels:

Consider making any required dietary changes and monitoring your blood sugar in accordance with your doctor's advice.

5. Reliable Mealtime Routine:

To help control blood sugar levels, keep a regular eating routine.

Planning ahead and making informed decisions can help you effectively manage a pregnancy with particular nutritional needs. It's essential to put your health and the health of your unborn child first by consulting with healthcare professionals and registered dietitians to develop a safe and balanced meal plan specific to your individual requirements, whether you are managing gestational diabetes, eating a vegetarian or vegan diet, need to avoid gluten or allergens, or are following a vegetarian or vegan diet.

Chapter 9: Postpartum Nutrition

Many congratulations on the birth of your child! Your nutritional requirements remain of the utmost significance as you move from pregnancy to the postpartum stage. The transition from pregnancy to postpartum, the foods that support recovery and breastfeeding, and meal planning for the fourth trimester a crucial period for both you and your baby are all topics covered in this chapter to help you through this special phase.

9.1 Pregnancy to Postpartum Transition

The time following childbirth is one of great physical and emotional change. Your body underwent a number of changes during pregnancy to support the expansion and development of your unborn child. It is currently returning to its pre-pregnancy state. Here's everything you need to know:

1. Nutrient Recovery: Your body needs time to recuperate from the physical stresses of pregnancy and childbirth. Focus on nutrient-dense foods to aid in the healing process.

2. Hormonal Adjustments: Hormonal changes continue after childbirth, affecting various bodily functions. Maintaining a balanced diet can help regulate these shifts.

3. Emotional Well-being: The postpartum period can be emotionally challenging. A healthy diet can support your mental well-being, ensuring you have the energy and emotional resilience to care for your new born.

9.2 Foods to Support Recovery and Breastfeeding

Proper nutrition during the postpartum period is crucial, especially if you're breastfeeding. Here are foods that can aid in recovery and support breastfeeding:

1. Lean Proteins: Protein-rich foods like lean meats, poultry, fish, and plant-based sources like beans and tofu help repair tissues and support milk production.

2. Calcium: Dairy products or fortified dairy alternatives are essential for maintaining strong bones and teeth. Calcium is also present in leafy greens and fortified cereals.

3. Iron: Iron is necessary to replenish the blood lost during childbirth. Foods like lean beef, beans, lentils, and fortified cereals are good sources.

4. Omega-3 Fatty Acids: Omega-3 fatty acids found in fatty fish, flaxseeds, and walnuts can help reduce inflammation and support mood stability.

5. Fiber: Adequate fiber intake from whole grains, fruits, and vegetables can aid in digestion and prevent constipation, which is common postpartum.

6. Hydration: Staying well-hydrated is vital for both recovery and breastfeeding. Aim to drink plenty of water throughout the day.

9.3 Meal Planning for the Fourth Trimester

The postpartum period is often referred to as the "fourth trimester" because it's a time of significant adjustment for both you and your baby. Meal planning during this phase can make a world of difference. Here's how to approach it:

1. Make It Easy: Preparing meals in advance, or relying on prepared meal services, can be a lifesaver during those early weeks of sleepless nights and frequent feedings.

2. Nutrient-Rich Snacks: Stock up on healthy snacks like nuts, dried fruits, yogurt, and whole-grain crackers to keep your energy levels stable.

3. Balanced Meals: Continue to focus on balanced meals with lean proteins, whole grains, and plenty of fruits and vegetables. This will provide you with the nutrients you need for recovery and breastfeeding.

4. Support System: Don't hesitate to lean on your support system for help with meal preparation and household chores. Having nutritious meals available can reduce stress and support your recovery.

5. Consult with a Dietitian: If you have specific dietary concerns or restrictions, consider consulting with a registered dietitian who can provide personalized guidance.

The postpartum period is a time of physical and emotional transformation. Nourishing your body with nutrient-dense foods can help you recover and provide the essential nutrition required for successful breastfeeding. By planning your meals and seeking support from healthcare providers, you can embrace this time of growth and bonding with your newborn with confidence.

Chapter 10: Recipes for Baby's First Foods

Your child's nutritional demands change as they develop. This chapter will introduce you to the idea of baby-led weaning, give you recipes for homemade baby food, and walk you through the exciting process of starting your baby on solid foods.

10.1 Overview of Baby-Led Weaning

A method of introducing solid foods called "baby-led weaning" lets your infant take the initiative. It promotes self-feeding and the investigation of various flavors and textures. Here are some essential guidelines:

- Baby-led weaning normally starts at around six months old, when your baby can sit up un assisted and exhibit an interest in eating.

- Safe Foods: Start with ripe bananas, cooked sweet potato sticks, or avocado slices that are soft and simple to hold.

- Safety first: To avoid choking risks, always watch over your baby while they are eating. Eat nothing that is round, hard, or tiny.

- Gradually offer a range of foods, such as fruits, vegetables, grains, and proteins, as part of the progression.

- Continue breastfeeding or formula feeding in addition to solid foods to make sure your baby is receiving the vital nutrients they require.

10.2 Recipes for homemade baby food

Here are some wholesome homemade baby food recipes to get your child's culinary career started

1. Avocado Mash (six months or more)

Smoothly mash ripe avocado. This creamy, nutrient-dense dish is full of good fats and is simple for infants to grasp.

2. Sweet potato fries (age 6+):

Bake sweet potatoes until tender after cutting into finger-sized sticks. These are great for helping your baby learn gripping and feeding itself.

3. Banana Oatmeal (six months or more):

To make a filling and simple-to-eat supper, combine mashed

banana with cooked blended oats.

4. Pureed butternut squash (6 months or older):

Butternut squash may be steamed and pureed to give your baby new flavors and critical vitamins and minerals.

5. Infant Rice Cereal (6 months and up):

For a straightforward, simple-to-digest first food, combine rice cereal with breast milk or formula

6. Coins made with steamed carrots (7+ months):

To make carrot coins tender but not mushy, steam them. Your infant can get practice picking them up and feeding her.

7. Mashed peas (7 months or older):

Peas are a colorful, nutrient-rich dish that may be cooked and mashed. These are fantastic for enhancing fine motor abilities.

10.3 Introducing Solid Food to Your Baby

It's exciting to start your kid on solid foods. Here are some pointers to speed up the procedure:

1. Start Slowly: To rule out any potential allergies or sensitivities, start with one food at a time.

2. Provide Variety: Introduce a range of foods to broaden your baby's taste buds and promote a varied diet.

3. Keep an eye out for symptoms: Pay attention to your baby's signals. Do not compel them to eat if they turn away or appear uninterested. It's acceptable if not every dinner turns out well.

4. Increase in Texture: As your infant improves at chewing and swallowing, gradually move away from purees and toward more textured foods.

5. Continue Milk Feeds: Until your kid is about a year old, continue nursing or formula feeding in addition to solid foods.

6. Consistency is Key: To give your kid a feeling of structure, be consistent with mealtimes and daily schedules.

An important developmental milestone for your infant is when solid foods are introduced. Remember that both you and your child will learn from this experience as you enthusiastically embrace this adventure. You can help your baby get the nutrition they need for a healthy start on solid foods by using these homemade baby food recipes and advice.

About the Author

Dr. Adam C. stands as a beacon of inspiration in the fields of medicine, nutrition, and self-help, with a remarkable journey that exemplifies the transformative power of healthy living. Armed with a professional master's degree in health nutrition and years of experience, Dr. C. has become a guiding light for individuals seeking to embrace vibrant well-being and lead happier lives.

From an early age, Dr. C. navigated through a myriad of health challenges that ranged from genetic predispositions to the pitfalls of unhealthy eating. His personal struggle ignited a flame of determination within him, one that was fueled by the belief that the human body possesses an incredible ability to heal and rejuvenate through the right nourishment. Through steadfast dedication, Dr. C. managed to conquer his own ailments and emerged as a living testament to the transformative potential of a well-balanced lifestyle.

What sets Dr. Adam C. apart is his rich tapestry of experiences, having been deeply immersed in groundbreaking research in health food and diet-related domains. His quest to uncover the hidden treasures of nutrients within our meals has led to groundbreaking revelations that empower individuals to extract the maximum benefit from their dietary choices. Dr. C.'s research has not only contributed to the scientific community but has also served as a roadmap for countless individuals striving to optimize their health.

However, it is not just Dr. C.'s academic prowess that has touched lives it is his unparalleled compassion and empathy that truly make him a beacon of hope. His personal journey of triumph over adversity infuses his guidance with an authentic understanding of the challenges his readers and patients face. Dr. C. doesn't just prescribe nutritional plans; he fosters a deep connection with his audience, instilling in them the confidence to embark on their own transformative journeys.

Dr. Adam C.'s holistic approach reaches beyond the confines of traditional medicine. His insights have translated into self-help resources that empower individuals to take charge of their wellness narrative. His words resonate on paper as they do in person, making his books not mere guides, but trusted companions on the path to vitality.

In the realm of health and nutrition, Dr. C. shines as a true luminary. His core strengths lie in his ability to synthesize complex scientific findings into practical, actionable advice that individuals from all walks of life can seamlessly integrate into their routines. Dr. C.'s legacy is not just a collection of breakthroughs; it is a testament to the extraordinary potential that lies within each of us to overcome obstacles and embrace a life brimming with health, happiness, and fulfillment.

As an experienced doctor, passionate nutritionist, and empathetic author, Dr. Adam C. continues to transform lives, showing us that the journey to a healthier, happier existence is within our grasp, waiting to be unlocked through the power of informed choices and unwavering determination.